NATURAL HAIR BREAKAGE

How To Retain Length and Grow Long Healthy Afrocentric Hair

Argena Hall

ww.ShopAnegra.com

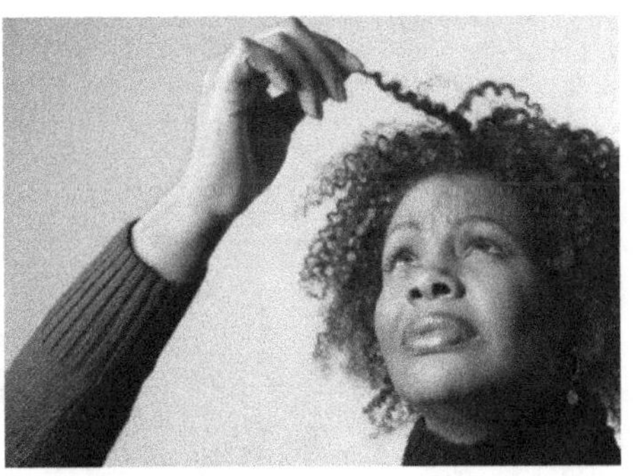

Table of Contents

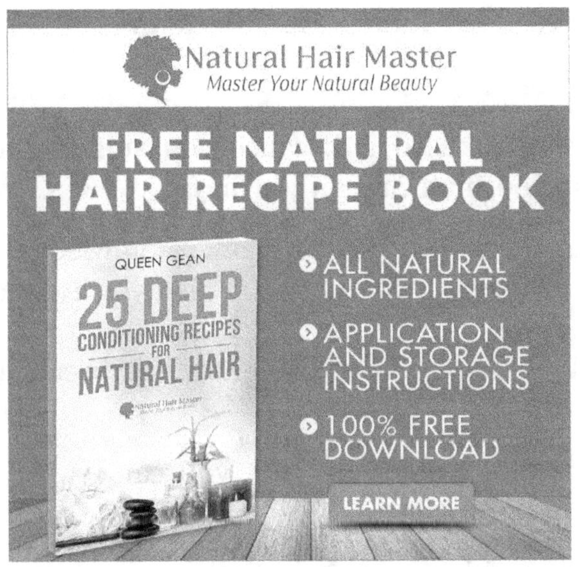

Visit **https://shopanegra.com/freerecipes** for your Deep Conditioning eBook!

Introduction

Thank you for reading *Natural Hair Breakage*!

You may have purchased it because you suffered from breakage (like myself) in your natural hair journey.

Or, you're just trying to garner as much knowledge about healthy hair care. Whichever is the reason, I'm glad you are today.

In this book, I will be breaking down how hair breakage happens.

As well as tips and techniques that you can employ in your hair regimen to help you with that.

This book will provide you with all the information needed to solve your hair breakage issues.

As well as, allowing your hair to reach an optimally healthy condition.

So grab a cup of tea, water, or juice and get reading!

CHAPTER 1: What is BREAKAGE?

Hair breakage as the term suggests is when your hair breaks apart.

It can break from the root, the middle of your hair strand, or even your ends.

Breakage should not be confused with shedding. Shedding of your natural hair is very normal.

You shed approximately 100 hairs per day. However, breakage is not shedding.

Breakage occurs because there is something wrong

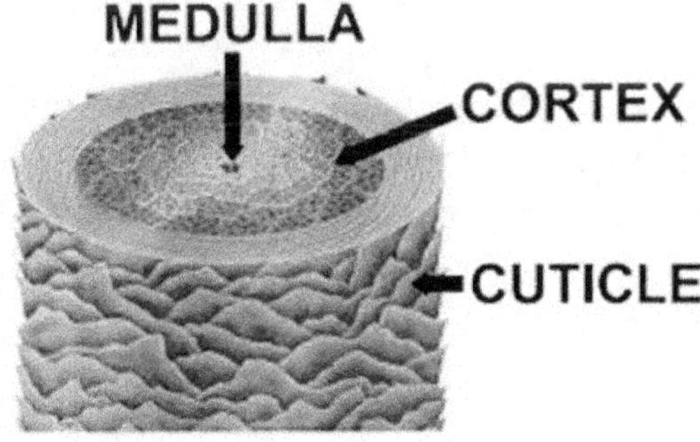

with your hair.

The hair has a protective layer on each strand called the cuticle. This cuticle protects the hair from any form of damage that is attacking the hair strand.

The cortex is made up of 90% protein, specifically keratin. It acts as a barrier and protects the hair from any form of damage.

Although it protects the hair, it can also be broken down, worn out, or neglected altogether.

Thus, making it easier for the hair strand to be attacked through various products and techniques. Therefore, causing our hair to break ... apart.

There are various reasons for breakage that are divided into three categories which are:
1. Mechanical; 2. Chemical; and 3. Environmental

1. MECHANICAL — Mechanical damage occurs from the daily, weekly, or monthly maintenance of our tresses. For example, we can be using products that offer no nutritional value to our hair. So, the hair is always in a dry state.

Once it gets to this point, it will cause a lot of friction amongst your hair strands. They will start rubbing against each other and forming knots, tangles, and "breaking apart". As well as, our techniques are not done in a manner that shows love and care for our mane.

We could be using a fine-tooth comb instead of a wide-tooth comb to detangle. And as such the fine teeth get stuck between the complex curly, coily or kinky nature of our curls. Thus, resulting in knots, tangles, and "breakage".

Hence, mechanical damage it as a result of the tools and products that we use for the maintenance of our hair.

2. CHEMICAL – Chemical damage occurs as a result of applying different chemical treatments to your hair. This could be from box dyes, lyes, bleach, hair-softening treatments, and much more. These "treatments" are damaging the health of your hair strand.

The hair has a protective layer on each strand called the cortex. This cortex protects the hair from any form of damage. The hair has a ph. range of 4 to 5. And often enough these "treatments" have a PH of 13, 14, and even 15. This means that they are in the alkaline region of the PH scale. So, they can chemically alter the structure of your hair strand to no return.

It can cause permanent damage that is difficult to repair. This is the reason why after using certain dyes our curls will go from tight to loose or kinky to completely straight. And as such, we recommend avoiding these chemicals that are doing nothing for the health of your hair.

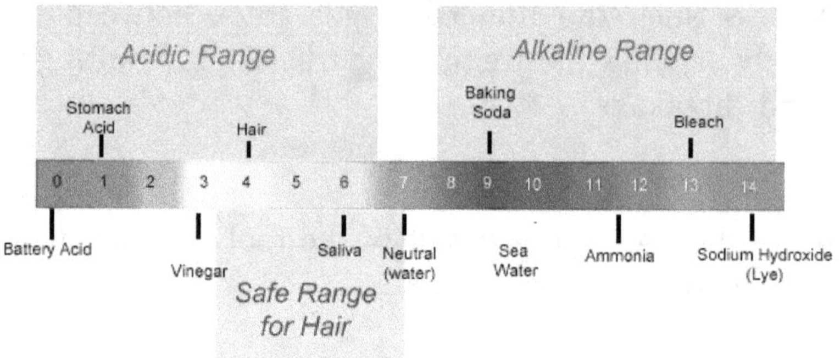

3. ENVIRONMENTAL – And finally is due to environmental damage. This is mainly due to the elements of the environment that we really and truly have no control over. For example, the sun shines daily, depending on the region of the world that you are in.

Those sun rays can penetrate the cuticle layer of the hair strand and cause some form of damage. And as the time gets even hotter, humid, or warmer, it can cause even more damage. As well as, our curls can be damaged from the saltwater content in our favorite water bodies (pools, beaches, creeks, etc).

The saltwater falls on the ph. scale between 9 and 10. Therefore, they have some effect on the health of your hair strands. It may strip the natural dark color of your hair strands and give you the "bleached" look. As well as, it can loosen the natural coily/kinky/curly pattern of your tresses.

Although we can recommend you avoid water bodies and stay out of the sun, it's not realistic. You may want to go to the beach with your friends or family or must run a quick errand on the road.

Therefore, we recommend protecting your hair when doing the activities that will have your air interacting with the environment for an extended period. See Chapters 3 and 4 for more information.

CHAPTER 2: SIGNS OF BREAKAGE

Depending on when you are along your natural hair journey, you may have or will experience breakage at least once.

If you are new to the natural hair community, you may hit that hurdle sooner than you expected if you are not aware of how to maintain the health of your hair.

Or, if you've been in the game for a long time, you may have made a misstep along your journey. And as such, the lack of knowledge or care will cause more harm than good to the health of your hair.

How to Identify A Broken Hair Strand:

This is important to know in your hair journey because as previously mentioned we can confuse shedding with breakage and vice versa. However, there is a distinct difference between the two. And that is if there is a bulb.

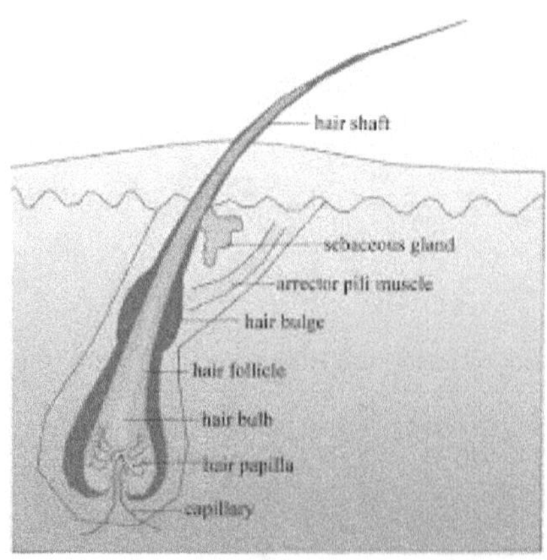

As per the diagram, the bulb is connected to the capillaries (aka the blood vessels). Once the vessels receive the nutrients from our blood it provides it to the scalp for our hair to grow. The first area of acceptance is the bulb.

So, the hair strand starting point is the bulb. Once you see a strand laying on the floor, wrapped up in the teeth or bristles of your comb or brush, look at it "KEENLY".

If you notice that the hair strand has a bulb at either end of it, then you are shedding.
If not, then my dear your natural hair is breaking.

And if you need more convincing,
then here are 10 signs that your hair may be breaking:

1. You see small hairs on your bedroom/bathroom floor –
This usually occurs when you are combing your hair into one of your favorite styles.

2. Your hair feels weak –
After touching your hair on wash or non-wash days, your hair feels weak, limp, or brittle.

3. You see small hairs on the bathroom sink –
This usually occurs when if you re detangling in your bathroom over the sink.

4. Your hair always feels dry (especially the ends) –
On non-wash days, your hair strand and ends always feel dehydrated and in need of moisture.

5. You see small hairs on your clothes after a day –
After a day of running errands, going to work, or just staying inside, you notice small broken pieces of your hair on your clothes.

6. You see clumps of broken hair strands when you are detangling –
When detangling your hair on wash days you see clumps of "short" hair strands falling out or on the comb/brush.

7. Your hair strands, especially the ends, look uneven when rocking certain hairstyles –
Your wash and go have varying degrees of short and long pieces.

8. Your hair isn't elastic anymore, so it doesn't curl like it used to –
When you stretch your curls and let it go, it doesn't quickly snap back into its natural curl pattern.

9. Your hair is more tangled –
Detangling your hair has become harder and more time-consuming.

10. Your hair doesn't feel like it usually does after certain treatments –
Your hair doesn't feel soft, nourished, moisturized, or strong after certain healthy hair treatments.

CHAPTER 3: HOW TO PREVENT BREAKAGE

Now that we know the causes of breakage as well as how to identify it, we need to know how to prevent it. There is a saying that says "prevention is better than cure" which holds true to this day.

We can employ steps within our natural hair regimen needed to prevent (correct or even reduce) the breakage that our hair is suffering from. And the best way is to ensure that our hair has the "moisture-protein" balance.

Our hair needs to have a balance of both moisture and protein for it to function in an optimal condition. It always needs to stay hydrated with various moisturizing treatments.

As well as, the cuticle layer needs to be strengthened with various protein treatments. This will prevent anything from attacking the hair strands, causing moisture to be lost, leaving the hair strand dry and susceptible to damage.

MOISTURE

Naturally, our hair strand is dry because the sebum that is produced by our scalp is not able to travel from the roots of our hair to the ends. It usually gets stuck in between the corners and crevices of our curl patterns.

Therefore, you usually feel your scalp and the hair's closest to it feeling greasy. That grease is called sebum which is filled with minerals that the hair needs. The sebum is produced by the blood vessels that transport vital minerals to the various areas of the body (including the scalp).

Naturally, the sebum should coat the entire hair strand and provide it with what it needs as it would straighter hair since this doesn't happen, we must take moisturizing our hair into our hair hands.

This is usually done in the form of conditioning, deep conditioning, and doing the LOC Method.

Conditioning: After shampooing, you should condition your tresses. The conditioner contains ingredients that should replenish your hair with the moisture that lost during the shampoo process. Therefore, most hair care experts recommend that you use shampoo and conditioner from the same brand. Manufacturers have created the products to work best with each other. Conditioners contain fatty alcohol that aid in providing the hair with the moisture that it needs. It can penetrate the hair strand to feed it with the minerals needed to not only moisturize. It will soften, add shine as well as enhance your natural curl pattern.

Deep Conditioning: Then, you rinse and follow up with your deep conditioner. As a natural, there is no way you should be missing out on deep conditioning your tresses (unless there is an emergency of course). Deep conditioner is one of the key steps in your natural hair regimen. Deep conditioners are made with natural ingredients that can fortify your hair strands. Therefore, it will penetrate to the deepest layer to provide the hair strand with moisture and protein that it needs. Some naturals have even credited deep conditioning for reviving the health of their lifeless curls. And you can too!

LOC (or LCO) Method:

And finally is to do the LOC Method.

The LOC method is one of the best moisturizing techniques for our hair because it does what a lot of others can't. Once the hair is provided with moisture that it needs, it is then sealed into the hair tresses. The sealing is important because it allows the moisture to be locked into the hair strands for a long time. This is usually until the next wash day or for the duration of your hairstyle.

The acronym stands for:

LIQUID – The first step is to apply Liquid (aka water) to your hair. Similarly to how plants love water, so does our hair.

Water offers our hair the best hydration that it needs. The h2o molecules will attach to the hair strand penetrate it and cause it to swell. This is usually when your curls start to form.

Examples of Liquids to Use:

1. Water,
2. Aloe Vera Juice,
3. Or a Water-Based Moisturizer.

OIL – The next step is to apply oil.

The oil is the first step of the sealing process. If you remember from middle school, water and oil do not mix. So, if they are in the same test tube, the oil will find its way on top of the water. It will sit there and prevent the water from escaping.

Similarly, to how it works for science, it works the same way on our hair. The oil will trap the h2o molecules unto the hair strand and prevent the hydration from leaking. Ensure to apply the oil using the praying hands' method to ensure that the oil is evenly coated on each strand.

Examples of Oils to Use:
1. Olive
2. Coconut
3. Rosehip
4. Grapeseed
5. Almond
6. Jojoba
and so much more.

CREAM – And finally you apply your favorite cream.
The cream is the last sealant that just holds everything in together in and on your hair strands. The butter/cream that you use will

keep the hydration from the liquid locked in as well as any additional benefits from your chosen oil.

As well as, the butter/cream will provide the hair strands with additional minerals as well.

Examples of Creams to Use: Cupuachu, Carrot, Grapeseed, and Shea Butter.
With all these ways, your curls are always staying hydrated.
Thus, reducing the likelihood if your curls become dry and susceptible to breakage.

PROTEIN:

You should also ensure that your hair is getting enough protein treatments as well. Our hair strands are made-up pf 90% protein, specifically keratin.

As previously mentioned, this aids in keeping the outer layer of hair strands thick, strong, and healthy. So, they can withstand against any future damage that's coming their way. If your hair isn't getting enough protein, then it becomes weak and/or brittle. Thus, making it more susceptible to being damaged.

So, we must do protein treatments. Protein treatments provide our hair with the protein that it needs ever so often to repair, build, and strengthen the hair strand. We recommend doing a protein treatment every 4 to 6 weeks in your hair regimen.

Example of protein Treatment: Monthly treatments using your favorite protein conditioner or a DIY Protein Treatment (using gelatine or eggs).

Now that we know how to prevent breakage, let's learn about how to retain our length.

CHAPTER 4: How to Retain Length

A misconception that a lot of naturals have is that my hair does not grow.
However, your hair does grow, it is always growing.
Studies have shown that hair grows on average ½ inch a month.

And, depending on your genetics if you are mixed with Caucasian (or Indian) it will grow even more than that. So the question you are asking yourself is, "so why am I not seeing it?"

You are not seeing it because you are not retaining your length.
So while your hair is growing and growing, the ends are breaking.
So as you grow you lose some.
So, you must implement steps in your hair regimen to aid in your length retention.

Here are 8 key steps to length retention:

1. **Detangling When Your Hair is Wet** – You should only detangle your hair when it is in a wet (or damp) state. Remember water makes your hair curl up because the strands are absorbing the water.

   Therefore, it makes it more pliable and easier to handle. So, it is recommended to detangle your hair when it is in this state. The comb, brush or your fingers can glide through the curl easier without causing any friction, tangles or knots.

Also, it is even better to detangle with conditioner or deep conditioner in your hair. We already discussed the benefits of conditioning and deep conditioning your hair in relation to breakage.

However, both products contain the key ingredient that gives the conditioning agent the "slip" that we all know and love. It called "Cetearyl alcohol". If your conditioning agent doesn't have it, then you need to get the next one. Cetearyl alcohol is a form of fatty alcohol that aids in softening the tresses, to make it more pliable and easier to handle for detangling.

2. **Use Satin-lined items** – Unlike cotton, satin doesn't take away the moisture that you worked so hard to put into your tresses. It acts as a barrier between the environment and your hair. Hence, it keeps the moisture locked in right where you put it. Therefore, satin is recommended whether you sleep on satin sheets, pillowcases, scarves, or with a satin cap.

   Once the moisture stays locked in, it maintains the hydration in our hair strands especially our ends. Thus, reducing the possibility of our hair becoming dry and susceptible to breakage.

3. **Moisturize using the LOC Method** – You can also moisturize your hair using the LOC Method. It is a moisture technique that keeps the moisture sealed into your hair strands for a long time to retain your hair length. The LOC method was discussed in detail in chapter 3, so refer to it for

the details.

4. **Wear Satin Clothing** – This tip goes hand in hand with number 2. We recommend wearing satin clothing if your hair is going to be out and about. If the hair encounters your clothes there will be no friction. No friction meaning no tangles, knots, and more importantly no breakage. Thus, aiding in allowing you to retain hair length.

5. **Keep Your Hair Tangle Free** – If your hair is not able to get tangles, then there will be no reason for friction. Friction causes our hair to rub against each other and form knots and tangles.

   Hence, we must avoid it all costs. So, keeping your hair tangle-free by keeping your hair in a stretched state. For example, when washing your hair keep your hair in 2, 4, or even 6 sections. This will prevent the hair from tangling up with each other. You can use section clips, or d loose twist/ braids to keep the sections separated. As well as, you can low manipulation (#6) or protective styling (#7).

6. **Wear Low Manipulation Styles** – Or, you can rock low manipulation styles. Low manipulation styles as the name suggest are styles that require little to no maintenance. So, once you style, you don't have to do much to it until a couple of days or until your wash days.

   Thus, keeping your hands out of your hair and reducing the friction, over manipulation, moisture loss and so much. And therefore, reducing the possibility of breakage.

Examples of Low-Manipulation Styles: Braid/Twist Outs, Buns, Crown Braids, Low Ponytail, Wash and Go.

7. **Wear Protective Styles** – As well as, you can choose to wear protective styles. Protective styles aid in length retention because they "protect" your natural hair. The synthetic hair wraps around your natural hair and prevents moisture loss, knots, and most importantly breakage.

    So, you will be reducing breakage, boosting length retention as well as rocking a new hairstyle.
    Examples of Protective Styles: Knotless Braids, Havanna Braids/Twists, Marley twists, Crochet Braids/Twists, Mini Twists/Braids, and much more.

8. **Doing consistent protein treatments** – Remember protein treatments are necessary for the health of your hair. Protein treatments were discussed in detail in Chapter 3.

Retaining your length is not an overnight process.
You must be consistent with the steps previously mentioned for you to see your true length results.

CHAPTER 5: TIPS FOR HEALTHY NATURAL HAIR

Now that we've discussed breakage, length retention, and much more.
Let's talk about simple hair tips that you can do to maintain the health of your hair.

There are changes in your hair's regimen and lifestyle that you can do. These will promote hair growth, maintain moisture levels, aid in length retention, add shine, and enhance the definition of your curls.

1. CUT YOUR HAIR (WHEN NECESSARY) – Yes, cut your hair.
Your hair ends go through a lot form styling, rubbing against your clothes, in other's people's hands and so much more. No wonder it's weathered, dry, not curling, tangled up, splitting and so much more.

When your ends get to this state, cut it. Let your dead irreparable ends go so that the healthy hair can thrive. For example, if you cut your split ends it prevents them from splitting from the ends right up to the root. And causing damage to the follicle layer for each strand. So, cut it naturalista.

You don't have to a major cut, for example cutting 6 inches off when you only had 1 inch of damage. Dust your hair ends as you see necessary. If you see split ends and single strand knots that are causing more harm than good, cut it off.

Do not be afraid to cut your hair. As previously mentioned, your hair is always growing so it will grow back. Once you cut it, you leave your ends in a healthier state. So, you twist or braid out will look better, your wash and go will curl more, and your hair will be easier to style into a bun.

2. TAKE VITAMINS – Take your vitamins daily as well.
While we do recommend eating a balanced diet every day, 3 times a day, you will not get all the minerals that the body needs. And as such, vitamins come into play here. They provide the body with those extra key ingredients that it needs to fully function.

Ensure to contact your family physician before deciding to take any of these items. The medical professional can tell you what to take best on your age, weight, pre-existing health conditions, and much more.

Examples of vitamins/supplements:
-fish oil
-omegas
-folates
-biotin
-vitamin b
-vitamin c
-and much more.

3. USING AYURVEDIC HERBS – Use Ayurveda herbs in your natural regimen.

Ayurveda is a practice in which you use natural herbs form the environment to heal your mind and body. It has been used for centuries by individuals from eastern societies or of eastern descent.

These herbs are used in their families in their food, on their bodies, in their hair, and have become a part of their overall lifestyle. The use and benefits of the herbs have been passed down from generations. They have attributed the health, length, and sheen of their hair to these same herbs.

And such, it has been adopted in the natural hair community because these herbs bring the hair to its optimum point. Even well-known brands have adopted some of these herbs in their products and utilize it is as a selling point.

Why? Because the plants aid in repairing the hair strands to bring it to the best state. The plants can be used in the form of herbs or oils. They can be added to your favorite hair products such as shampoos, conditioners, or deep conditioners.

They will boost the properties of each product for it to boost the overall health of your hair. Luckily these herbs are easily accessible and can be purchased on Amazon or at your local beauty supply store.

Examples of oils:
1. Shikakai
2. Bhringaraj
3. Brahmi
4. Neem
5. Amla
6. Henna

7. Hibiscus
8. Fenugreek
and much more.

4. Exercise Daily – Exercising is another activity to implement into your regimen, that allows your blood to stay pumping. Remember we want our blood to continually flow to provide the scalp with the minerals that it needs.

Hence, we recommend exercising daily for 15 minutes. The form of exercise doesn't matter if you get your body moving. You can go ride bikes, take a walk, dance, swim, lift weights, track and so many more exercises.

5. Protect Your Hair from The Sun – While vitamin D is good for the body, it may not necessarily be good for your hair. The UV light rays coming from the sun are strong in their chemical element. They can penetrate the hair shaft and cause more harm than good to it. If you are frequently outside in the sun, the light rays can break down the protective layer of your hair strands.

Therefore, making it more susceptible to damage from additional light rays, the environment, products, and tools that we use. Hence, we recommend if you're going to be in the sun for an extended period, wear a hat or scarf. It will block the light rays from penetrating your hair shaft.

6. No Chemical Dyes on Your Hair – Our hair has a protective layer that is made up of protein. That layer is there to maintain the health of your strands from any form of damage.

However, it can break down my significant heat penetration from the sun, hot tools as well as chemicals in our hair products. The commercial dyes are made with a high chemical compound that usually falls within the alkaline side of the PH scale. Therefore, they can alter the genetic makeup structure of our hair strands.

7. MASSAGE YOUR SCALP – Massage your scalp daily.
Scalp massages aid in promoting healthy hair growth. Massaging your scalp helps to promote blood circulation beneath the scalp. The blood is the transport system of the body.

So, the vitamins from the foods (#4) and vitamins (#5) that we take, will be transported via the blood to the various areas of the blood. The bulb (see chapter 2) will absorb the minerals from the blood via the blood vessels needed to feed the scalp, the scalp will produce sebum in the bulb for it to coat our new growth.

And as such, scalp massages not only contribute to hair growth, but it allows sebum production for that hair growth as well. So as new hairs are being produced, they are being nourished so they can withstand against any future damage. Inverting your head while doing scalp massages allows the blood to flow faster the scalp for faster hair growth.

In addition, use essential oils while massaging your scalp.

Essential oils contain antifungal, antiviral, antibacterial, antiseptic, and antimicrobial properties. These can fight off the free radicals that are beneath the scalp that are wreaking havoc on your healthy hair journey.

These radicals are causing psoriasis, slow growth, alopecia, itchy and inflamed scalp. The oils soothe the scalp by stopping the formation of these free radicals. Thus, allowing the scalp to function in a normal and optimum manner. Ensure to use these essential oils with carrier oils.

Essential oils are so potent and rich that they cannot be used on the scalp alone. If they are, they may burn it. Therefore, you should mix them with a carrier to "dilute" it so it's safer for the scalp.

Examples of Essential Oils:
-Rosemary Oil
-Tea tree Oil
-Lavender Oil
-Lemon Oil
-Peppermint Oil
-Lemongrass Oil
-Orange Oil
-and Eucalyptus Oil.

8. EAT HEALTHY– A balanced diet is important for the health of our body.
More so important for the health of our hair. Did you know that the nutrients you consume daily go to your skin, nails, and hair last?

Yes, that's correct. So, if you are eating junk food that has little to no nutritional value, then your hair will suffer. Therefore, you need to eat a balanced diet 3 times a day. Your diet should consist of carbs, protein, vegetables, fruits, and water.

The foods from these various food categories are rich in minerals, vitamins, and other nutrients that your hair will thank you for later.

Side Note: If you want your hair to be longer, stronger and thicker, ensure that the diet is rich in protein. Remember the hair strand is made up of keratin (a form of protein). So, if we are eating the protein consistently, the body will convert the protein to keratin when it is transporting it via the blood system to the scalp. Therefore, eat lots of protein.

Examples of protein-rich foods are:
-Eggs,
-Chicken Breast
-Salmon
-Fish,
-Nuts
-Legumes
and much more.

9. Avoid Heat Styling – Similarly to the heat from the sun, the heat from hot tools will do just about, less or more damage to your hair strands. Hot tools include flat irons, curling irons, blow dryers, and others.

We suggest doing no heat styling whatsoever to preserve the life of your hair strands. However, if you can't avoid then we recommend using a "good" heat protectant. It will act as a protective barrier between your hair strands and the heat from the tools.

10. Cleansing Your Scalp - A healthy scalp is a start for healthy hair.
If your scalp is not in a healthy condition, neither will the rest of your hair be.

Your scalp goes through a lot as products are being applied to it, sebum is being produced, and different elements of the environment are attaching itself to it. All of these can block the scalp's follicles and prevent it from breathing.

As well as, allow for bacteria and dirt to fester on the scalp and harbor your growth process and sebum production. And as such, you should be cleansing your scalp every week.

Cleansing with a sulfate-free shampoo allows your scalp to be thoroughly cleansed without removing the "natural sebum from your scalp". Hence, your hair will not be dry as it is being cleansed which can lead to more damage.

CONCLUSION

Now that you know what to do solve, prevent, repair or reduce your hair breakage,
DO IT!

You have the knowledge needed to allow your hair to flourish so get started.
I hope you were taking notes while reading this book.

This book was created to serve you by allowing you to learn about your hair to solve its hair issues. Thus, allowing you must stronger, healthier, thicker, and shinier natural hair.

Lastly, if you enjoyed this book, please consider leaving a review. Leaving a review will help others to find our books and gives us feedback on how we can improve the book.

Thanks again for your support. I wish you all the best in your journey. God Bless!

Check Out My Other Books

Below you'll find some of my other natural hair books.

Natural Hair Growth Secrets

The Beginners Guide To Natural Hair

Natural Hair Recipes

Shampoo Making

The Big Chop

Natural Hair Transitioning

Visit **www.ShopAnegra.com** for our newest books, journals, and beauty supplies!

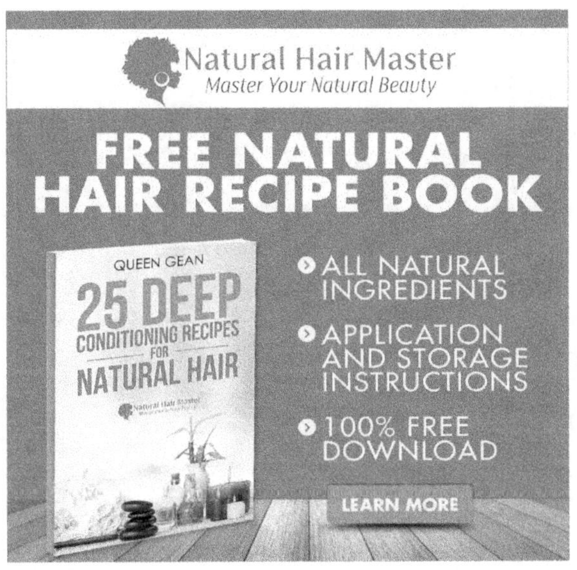

Visit **https://shopanegra.com/freerecipes** for your Deep Conditioning eBook!